QUICKLY LOSE

BELLY FAT

GREAT ASSISTANCE AND HEALTHY FOODS TO HELP MELTS FAT

By

Gerald J. Blake

Disclaimer

All may be reproduced, distributed, or transmitted in any form or by any means, including photocopying, recording, or other electric or mechanical method, without the prior written permission of the publisher, except in the case of brief quotations embodied in critical review and certain other noncommercial uses permitted by copyright law. Copyright© Gerald J. Blake.

TABLE OF CONTENTS

INTRODUCTION

Getting rid of abdominal fat is a problem that many people encounter. But there are rules to follow, as well as foods that can lower amounts of belly fat and overall body fat and meals that can do the opposite.

Why not add it to your basket after scrolling up to learn more about it? The book covers food items that increase abdominal fat. foods that aid in abdominal fat reduction or fat dissolution.

Without causing stress, these methods quicken the process of losing belly weight.

CHAPTER ONE

The chance of developing several chronic illnesses may increase if you have too much belly fat. You can reduce belly fat by cutting back on alcohol consumption, increasing your protein intake, and doing weights.

Having too much belly fat can harm your health and increase your risk of developing several chronic illnesses.

Visceral fat, a particular type of belly fat, is a significant contributor to the risk of type 2 diabetes, heart disease, and other diseases.

Body mass index (BMI) is used by several health organizations to categorize weight and determine the likelihood of developing metabolic diseases.

BMI, however, only accounts for height and weight and ignores body composition or visceral fat.

There are several things you can do even though losing fat in this area can be challenging.

I. THERE ARE 18 EFFICIENT WEIGHT-LOSS STRATEGIES

1. Consume a lot of soluble fiber.

The gel that is created when soluble fiber absorbs water assists digestion by slowing down the passage of food.

According to studies, this fiber may make you feel fuller, which will cause you to eat less naturally.

And soluble fiber might also aid with abdominal fat loss.

With every 10-gram (g) increase in soluble fiber intake, belly fat accumulation fell by 3.7% over five years, according to an older observational study involving more than 1,100 adults.

Vegetables, fruits, beans, oats, barley, and legumes are excellent sources of soluble fiber.

In summary, you might lose weight by consuming more soluble fiber, which also makes you feel fuller while consuming fewer calories. Make an effort to consume a lot of high-fiber foods.

2. Steer clear of foods with trans fats.

By injecting hydrogen into unsaturated fats like soybean oil, trans fats are produced.

They used to be included in various kinds of margarine and spreads and were frequently added to packaged goods, but the majority of food companies no longer use them.

In observational and animal research, these lipids have been connected to inflammation, heart disease, insulin resistance, and belly fat growth.

In a 6-year study, it was discovered that monkeys that consumed more trans-fat developed 33% more belly fat than those who consumed more monounsaturated fat.

Read ingredient labels closely and avoid using products that contain trans fats to help reduce belly fat. These are frequently labeled as partially hydrogenated fats.

A high trans-fat intake has been associated with increased belly fat gain, according to some research. Limiting your intake of trans fat is a good notion whether or not you're trying to lose weight.

3. Limit your alcohol consumption.

Alcohol can be good for your health in moderation, but excessive consumption can be detrimental.

According to research, drinking too much booze may increase belly fat.

Observational studies show a substantial rise in the chance of developing excess fat storage around the waist when heavy alcohol consumption occurs.

Alcohol consumption reduction may aid in weight loss. It's not necessary to stop, but cutting back on how much you consume each day can be beneficial.

Over 2,000 people participated in one research on alcohol consumption. According to the findings, those who drank alcohol regularly but on average only had one drink had less belly obesity than those who drank less frequently but more frequently on the days they drank.

The most current Dietary Guidelines for Americans state that men should limit their alcohol consumption to two drinks per day or less and women should limit their alcohol consumption to one drink per day or less.

In Summary, Abdominal fat has been found to rise with excessive alcohol consumption. If you're attempting to lose weight, think about consuming alcohol in moderation or not at all.

4. Consume a diet rich in protein.

For controlling weight, protein is a crucial substance.

A high-protein diet boosts the production of the hormone peptide YY, which suppresses hunger and encourages fullness.

Additionally, protein increases metabolic rate and aids in muscle retention during weight reduction.

Numerous observational studies reveal that individuals who consume more protein typically have less abdominal fat than those who consume less protein.

Make sure to include a quality protein source at every meal, such as meat, seafood, eggs, dairy products, whey protein, and beans.

In summary, if you're attempting to lose belly fat, eating foods high in protein, like seafood, lean poultry, and beans, may be helpful.

5. Lower your tension level

The adrenal glands' production of cortisol, also known as the stress hormone, is what causes worry to cause belly fat gain.

According to studies, high levels of cortisol cause appetite to rise and the storage of abdominal fat.

Women with large waists also tend to respond to worry by producing more cortisol. The accumulation of belly obesity is further exacerbated by elevated cortisol.

Play stress-relieving games to aid in abdominal fat loss. It may be beneficial to practice yoga or meditation.

In summary. Your waistline could become fatter as a result of stress.

If you're attempting to lose weight, reducing stress should be one of your top priorities.

6. Avoid consuming a lot of sugary meals.

When consumed in excess, fructose has been related to several chronic diseases.

These consist of fatty liver illness, type 2 diabetes, and heart disease.

Observational studies demonstrate a link between excessive sugar consumption and increased belly fat.

Realize that other factors besides refined sugar can contribute to belly fat development. Even natural sugars, like true honey, ought to be consumed in restraint.

In summary, for many individuals, consuming too much sugar contributes significantly to weight gain. Reduce your consumption of candy and processed meals that contain added sugar.

7. Perform a cardio workout (cardio)

Cardiovascular exercise, or aerobic exercise, is a powerful method to enhance your health and burn calories.

It can be a useful type of exercise for shedding belly fat, according to studies. The effectiveness of mild versus high-intensity exercise is, however, debatable.

In any event, how frequently and how long you exercise can be very crucial.

According to one research, postmenopausal women lost more body fat from all areas when they engaged in aerobic activity for 300 minutes per week as opposed to 150 minutes per week.

However, researchers also pointed out that neither group's changes in visceral belly fat were substantially different from one other.

In summary, an efficient way to lose weight is through aerobic activity. Studies indicate it's especially effective at lowering body fat in general and belly fat in particular.

8. Limit carbohydrates, particularly refined carbohydrates.

Cutting back on carbohydrates can help you lose weight, including belly fat.

In reality, low-carb diets may help those who are overweight, at risk for type 2 diabetes or have polycystic ovary syndrome lose belly fat. (PCOS).

You don't have to adhere to a rigid low-carbohydrate diet. According to some studies, switching to unprocessed starchy carbohydrates instead of refined carbohydrates may benefit metabolic health and decrease belly fat.

According to the Framingham Heart Study, those who consumed the most whole grains had a 17% lower risk of having excess abdominal obesity than those who consumed the least.

In summary, Excessive belly obesity is linked to consuming a lot of refined carbohydrates. Think about cutting back on your consumption of refined carbohydrates or swapping them out for healthy carb sources like whole grains, legumes, or vegetables.

9. Carry out strength exercises (lift weights)

Exercises that build and maintain muscle mass include resistance training, also referred to as weightlifting or strength training.

Resistance training may also help with belly fat reduction, according to studies involving individuals with prediabetes, type 2 diabetes, and fatty liver disease.

A study involving overweight teens found that the largest reduction in visceral fat occurred when strength training and aerobic exercise were combined.

If you decide to start weightlifting, it's a good idea to consult a physician first and seek guidance from a licensed personal trainer.

In summary, Strength training can be a crucial weight reduction strategy and may reduce belly fat. According to studies, combining it with aerobic exercise makes it even more efficient.

10. Reduce the number of drinks with added sugar.

Frequent consumption of added sugars like fructose, which can increase belly fat, is common in drinks with added sugars.

One study on individuals with type 2 diabetes discovered that drinking at least one serving of sugar-sweetened beverages each week was linked to more belly fat than drinking less than one serving each week.

Furthermore, since your brain doesn't handle liquid calories the same way it does solid ones, you might end up overeating later on and storing the excess calories as fat.

It's ideal to restrict your consumption of sugar-sweetened beverages, such as: • soda, to lose belly fat.

• booze mixers that contain sugar; punch; sweet tea;

In summary, if you're trying to reduce belly fat, it's crucial to keep your intake of liquid sugar, such as sugar-sweetened beverages, to a minimum.

11. Obtain a lot of sound slumbers.

Your health, including your weight, depends on sleep in many ways. According to studies, some individuals may be more at risk of becoming obese and developing more belly fat if they don't get enough sleep.

In a 16-year research involving over 68,000 women, it was discovered that those who slept for less than 5 hours each night had a significantly higher risk of gaining weight than those who slept for 7 hours or more.

Excess visceral fat has also been connected to the disease known as sleep apnea, where breathing stops periodically throughout the night.

Make sure you are receiving enough high-quality sleep in addition to sleeping for at least 7 hours every night.

Consider consulting a doctor about available treatments if you think you may have sleep apnea or another sleep problem.

In summary, a higher chance of weight gain has been associated with sleep deprivation. If you're attempting to lose weight, getting enough good sleep is crucial.

12. Monitor your diet and activity.

There are many ways to reduce your weight and abdominal fat, but the most important is to eat fewer calories than your body requires to maintain your weight.

You can keep track of your calorie consumption by keeping a food journal or by using an app or online food tracker. It has been demonstrated that this tactic helps people lose weight.

You can also see your intake of protein, carbohydrates, fiber, and micronutrients with the aid of meal-tracking tools. Many also let you keep track of your physical activity and workouts.

On this page, you can find several free applications or websites for tracking your calorie and nutrient consumption.

In summary, keeping a note of your meals can be beneficial if you're trying to lose weight. One of the most common methods to do this is by keeping a food journal or by using an online food tracker.

13. Regularly consume fatty seafood.

A balanced diet may benefit from including fatty seafood.

They are abundant in omega-3 fatty acids and high-quality protein, both of which may help to prevent chronic illness.

These omega-3 fats may also aid in the reduction of visceral fat, according to some data.

Omega-3 supplements may substantially reduce liver and abdominal fat, according to studies on adults and kids with fatty liver disease.

Each week, try to eat two to three portions of fatty fish. Good options include salmon, herring, sardines, mackerel, and anchovies.

Omega-3 supplements made from plants, such as algae, are also available for vegetarians, vegans, and people who don't typically eat seafood.

summary, consuming fatty seafood and supplementing with omega-3 fatty acids derived from fish oil or algae may both enhance general health. It may also help those with the fatty liver disease lose belly fat, according to some data.

14. Consume citrus juice in moderation

Fruit juice offers vitamins and minerals, but it frequently has sugar levels comparable to those of soda and other sweetened drinks.

For instance, there are 24 g of sugar, more than half of which is fructose, in an 8-ounce (248 milliliters) portion of unsweetened apple juice.

According to research, drinking a lot of fruit juice may cause weight gain because it includes an excessive number of calories rather than fructose.

However, you should limit your consumption and opt for other drinks with less sugar, like water, unsweetened iced tea, or sparkling water with a wedge of lemon or lime.

In summary, Fruit juice frequently has the same quantity of sugar as soda and, if consumed in large quantities, may cause weight gain. It's best to limit your consumption and indulge in other libations like water or unsweetened iced tea.

15. Consume probiotic cuisine or a probiotic dietary supplement.

In some meals and supplements, probiotics are bacteria. They might benefit your health in ways like boosting your immune system and promoting better digestive health.

The proper balance of bacteria, according to research, can aid in weight loss, including the reduction of belly fat. Different kinds of bacteria have been found to play a role in weight regulation.

The Lactobacillus genus, which includes strains like Lactobacillus fermentum, Lactobacillus amylovorus, and Lactobacillus gasseri, has been shown to help people lose belly fat.

Probiotics might help with weight loss, but more study is required. It's crucial to consult a doctor before including probiotics or other supplements in your regimen since some bacteria aren't governed by the Food and Drug Administration.

In summary, one way to support a healthy gut system is by taking probiotic supplements. Additionally, research points to the possibility that weight reduction may be aided by advantageous gut flora.

16. Take into account waiting between meals.

Concerning weight loss, intermittent fasting has lately gained a lot of popularity.

A cycle between food and fasting occurs in this eating habit.

Fasting for 24 hours once or twice a week is a common technique. Another involves consuming all of your food within an 8-hour window after 16 hours of fasting each day.

According to one study, protein pacing, which entails eating nutrient-dense meals spaced equally throughout the day, combined with intermittent fasting led to greater losses in body weight, total fat, and visceral fat than calorie restriction.

Keep in mind that earlier research suggests that intermittent fasting may harm women's blood sugar control but not men's.

 Even though some modified intermittent fasting techniques seem to be better choices, you should cease fasting right away if you experience any side effects.

Before attempting intermittent fasting or making other dietary changes, consult a doctor as well.

In summary, Intermittent fasting is a type of eating that varies between eating and fasting times. According to studies, it might be among the best methods for reducing abdominal fat and weight.

17. Take green tea.

Green tea is incredibly healthy to drink.

The antioxidant epigallocatechin gallate (EGCG) and caffeine in it both seem to speed up metabolism.

Several studies indicate that catechin EGCG may aid in abdominal fat reduction. If you drink green tea and work out at the same time, the impact might be enhanced.

Intriguingly, a review found that green tea may help people lose weight, particularly if they take it in doses of less than 500 milligrams per day for 12 weeks.

Another study found that drinking green tea regularly could help people lose weight and shrink their waistlines.

In summary, Regular consumption of green tea has been connected to weight loss, though more study is required. It works best when combined with exercise though, as it's presumably less effective when used alone.

18. Adjust your habits and use a variety of techniques

One of these actions might not have a significant impact on its own.

Combining various approaches may produce the best outcomes.

It's interesting to note that a lot of these strategies are typically connected to healthy living and a balanced diet.

To lose your belly fat and keep it off, you must make long-term behavioral changes.

Fat loss usually occurs as a natural side effect when you practice healthy habits, keep active, and limit your consumption of highly processed foods.

In summary, if you don't keep up a consistent diet and other living choices, losing weight and keeping it off may be challenging.

The final word

Lose abdominal fat, there are no quick fixes.

It always takes work, dedication, and persistence to lose weight.

You may reduce belly fat and enhance your general health by implementing some or all of the methods and lifestyle objectives covered in this piece.

CHAPTER TWO

I.   SIX EASY, SCIENCE-BACKED METHODS FOR REDUCING BELLY FAT

Adopting a healthy diet and regular exercise is the best method to lose belly fat. To keep you on schedule, it can also be beneficial to journal your daily meals.

One typical weight loss aim is to reduce belly fat. The storing of energy and the control of hormones are just two of the many roles that fat plays in your body. It's beneficial to have some bodily fat.

The abdominal region is primarily composed of two kinds of fat. Your skin's immediate undersurface is where subcutaneous fat is found. Your body, including the midsection, has this fat deposited all over it.

Visceral fat is the other form of fat that is present in your abdomen. Deeper within your body, this fat protects the organs in your belly by cushioning them. High levels of this fat have been associated with diseases like type 2 diabetes and cardiac disease, according to research.

Because of this, reducing extra visceral fat can have a positive impact on your health.

By using a tape measure to measure the area around your midsection, you can determine how much fat is in your abdominal region. Abdominal obesity is defined as measurements of 40 inches (102 cm) or more for males and 35 inches (88 cm) or more for women.

There is a widespread misconception that visceral or abdominal fat can be reduced using specific weight reduction techniques. There isn't currently a scientifically validated method to "spot reduce" fat in specific areas through diet or exercise.

Your entire body usually experiences weight increase or loss, but depending on the individual, different parts of your body may change first. Your genes most likely have an impact on your special design.

Healthy weight loss methods are your best option if you're trying to lose belly fat. Here are 6 scientifically proven methods for losing weight, including belly fat.

1. Avoid sugary and sugar-sweetened beverages.

Overweight abdominal obesity may result from a diet rich in added sugars.

According to studies, additional sugar specifically harms the health of the metabolic system.

Numerous studies have shown that excessive sugar, primarily because of the high fructose content, can cause fat to accumulate around your liver and belly.

Half of the sugar is fructose and half is glucose. The liver becomes overwhelmed with fructose when you consume a lot of added sugar and is compelled to convert it to fat.

Some people think that this is the primary mechanism causing sugar's detrimental impacts on health. It raises liver and abdominal fat, which can result in insulin resistance and several metabolic issues.

You might want to restrict liquid sugar in particular if you're attempting to cut calories. When you consume sugar-sweetened beverages, you end up eating more total calories because the brain doesn't seem to recognize liquid calories in the same way as solid calories.

A study found that every extra daily serving of sugar-sweetened beverages increased a child's risk of obesity by 60%.

Think about reducing the quantity of sugar in your diet and cutting back on sugar-sweetened beverages. This includes drinks with added sugar, sugary sodas, fruit juices, and different sports drinks with a lot of added sugar.

Make sure goods don't contain refined sugars by reading the labels. Even meals that are promoted as healthy can have sizable sugar content.

Remember that none of this pertains to whole fruit, which is very healthy and contains a lot of fiber, which counteracts the negative effects of fructose.

In summary, the main cause of extra fat in the liver and abdomen may be excessive sugar intake. This is especially valid for sweetened drinks.

2. Consume more proteins

For weight reduction, protein might be the most crucial macronutrient.

According to research, you can consume up to 441 fewer calories per day and experience a 60% reduction in cravings, an 80–100 calorie daily metabolism boost, and cravings.

The most successful dietary changes you can make if you want to lose weight include adding more protein to your diet.

Protein may be able to prevent you from gaining weight in addition to helping you drop it.

According to some data, eating more protein may result in less belly fat. According to one study, individuals with less abdominal fat ate more protein of higher quality.

According to different research, eating more protein is associated with women's waistlines expanding less over five years.

In addition, this research found a link between fruit and vegetable consumption and lower fat, and a link between refined carbs and oils and more belly fat.

Protein accounted for 25–30% of calories in many of the trials that found it helps people lose weight. So perhaps it would be wise to experiment with this spectrum.

By consuming more high-protein foods like whole eggs, fish, legumes, nuts, meat, and dairy goods, you can increase your consumption of protein.

You might think about incorporating a high-quality protein supplement to increase your overall intake if you have trouble obtaining enough protein in your diet. But before including any nutritional supplements in your regimen, consult your doctor.

Check out this piece for tips on how to eat more protein while on a vegetarian or vegan diet.

In summary, Protein is a very effective weight-loss strategy because it increases metabolism and curbs appetite. According to some data, eating more protein may result in less belly obesity.

3. Attempt a low-carb diet.

Losing weight can be accomplished by consuming very few carbohydrates or by adopting a ketogenic diet. These diets are not suitable for everyone, though, as they carry some possible risks.

Some people cut their daily carbohydrate intake to 50 grams if they want to drop weight quickly, which is significantly less than the average American diet's carbohydrate intake. Your body enters a state of ketosis as a result, where it begins to burn fat for energy.

When individuals cut out carbohydrates, their appetite usually decreases and they tend to lose weight.

Very low carbohydrate diets can occasionally result in weight reduction that is 2-3 times greater than that of low-fat diets, according to more than 20 randomized controlled studies.

This holds even when those in the low-carb groups are not calorie restricted but are instead permitted to consume as much as they please.

Not fat loss but decreases in water weight account for some of this weight loss. However, studies contrasting low-carb and low-fat diets show that low-carb eating particularly reduces belly fat.

This means that some of the fat lost on a low-carb diet is likely to be visceral fat, a type of abdominal fat that has been linked to health issues when present in large amounts.

In addition to helping people lose weight, low-carb diets can also have several positive health effects. For instance, they can greatly enhance the health of those who have type 2 diabetes.

Before beginning a very low-calorie or ketogenic diet, however, make sure to consult your doctor. If you have any health issues, this is particularly crucial.

On a restrictive diet like this one, it's a good idea to speak with a certified dietitian to make sure you're receiving all the nutrients you require.

In summary, Research indicates that reducing carbohydrate intake may be especially helpful in shedding abdominal fat. Consult your doctor before beginning a very low-carb regimen.

4. Take meals high in fiber.

Most dietary fiber is inedible plant debris.

Fiber consumption can aid in weight reduction. The sort of fiber, though, matters.

Your weight seems to be primarily influenced by soluble and thick fibers. The passage of food through your intestinal system can be significantly slowed down by this gel. The digestion and uptake of nutrients may also be slowed down. The outcome is a protracted sense of fullness and diminished appetite.

According to review research, an extra 14 grams of fiber per day was associated with a 10% reduction in caloric intake and a weight loss of about 4.5 pounds (2 kg) over 4 months.

Eating 10 grams of soluble fiber every day was associated with a 3.7% decrease in visceral fat in the abdominal cavity, according to 5-year research.

This suggests that soluble fiber might be especially useful for getting rid of the deeper abdominal fat that encircles your organs.

The best method to increase your fiber intake is to eat a lot of plant-based foods, such as fruit and vegetables. Additionally, some grains, like whole oats, and legumes are excellent sources.

Taking a fiber product like glucomannan is another option. Studies indicate that this dietary fiber, which is among the most vicious, may aid in weight reduction.

It's essential to consult your doctor before adding this or any other supplements to your diet.

In summary, there is some proof that soluble dietary fiber can cause abdominal fat levels to drop. Reducing excess visceral fat may enhance metabolic health and lower the chance of developing certain illnesses.

5. Consistently work out

One of the best things you can do to improve your odds of living a long, healthy life and avoiding illness is to exercise.

One of the incredible health advantages of exercise is that it can help decrease belly fat.

This does not preclude performing abdominal exercises, as spot reduction—losing fat in a specific area—is still feasible. In one trial, six weeks of abdominal-only exercise had no discernible impact on abdominal fat or waist circumference.

Both aerobic and weight training can help you lose body fat.

Visceral fat can be significantly reduced through aerobic activity, such as swimming, running, and walking.

Exercise appears to be especially crucial during weight maintenance, according to results of another study that showed it entirely prevented people from regaining visceral fat after weight loss.

Exercise can also help other metabolic issues like blood sugar control and inflammation reduction.

In summary, Exercise can be very beneficial for many different health conditions, including the reduction of visceral obesity in the abdomen.

6. Keep a dietary journal

Most people are aware that what you consume matters, but many are unaware of the specifics of what they're eating.

Without keeping track, it's simple to overestimate or underestimate one's food consumption, even if they believe they are following a high protein or low carb diet.

You don't have to weigh and measure every meal to keep track of your caloric consumption. If you want to lose weight by making dietary changes, keeping a note of your intake every so often for a few days can help you identify the most crucial areas for change.

Planning can assist you in achieving particular objectives, such as increasing your protein consumption to 25–30% of calories or reducing added sugars.

For a list of free online tools and apps to monitor what you're consuming, as well as a calorie counter, see these articles.

The final word

The organs in your abdomen are encircled by visceral fat. A higher chance of developing some health conditions is associated with having too much of it.

Most people can lose belly fat by making significant changes to their lifestyles, such as consuming a diet high in lean protein, vegetables, fruit, and legumes, and exercising frequently.

Before making significant changes to your eating or activity levels, it is essential to discuss them with your doctor if you have any medical conditions or a history of disordered eating. You can also get assistance from a certified dietitian to make sure that your diet plan is providing you with all the nutrition you require.

Check out this article on 26 scientifically proven weight reduction techniques for more weight loss advice.

II. THE TWO TYPES OF BELLY FAT AND HOW TO LOSE IT

Types of belly fat, Reasons why belly fat is unhealthy, Lose belly fat tips

It's common to have some belly fat. After all, adipose insulates and protects your body.

But having too much belly fat can be unhealthy and raise your chance of contracting some chronic illnesses. As a result, it can be beneficial to maintain a healthy amount of total body fat, including belly fat.

This article describes the different kinds of belly fat and offers evidence-based advice on how to get rid of extra belly fat.

What kinds of abdominal fat are there?

Only a tiny quantity of fat is found in your belly compared to the rest of your body.

One type of belly fat lies beneath your skin, and the other type is located deeper inside your abdomen, encircling your internal organs.

Subcutaneous abdominal fat

The fat beneath your epidermis is referred to as subcutaneous fat or subcutaneous adipose tissue (SAT).

Your belly's "jiggling" fat is subcutaneous fat, which is flexible. Generally speaking, women have more subcutaneous fat than males do.

Subcutaneous fat has a weaker association with increased disease risk than fat located deeper in the abdominal cavity.

The risk of getting some chronic diseases, such as type 2 diabetes, heart disease, and some cancers, may be increased by having too much body fat overall, including total belly fat.

On the other hand, preserving healthy levels of body fat all around and in your belly may lessen your chance of contracting a chronic illness.

abdominal visceral fat

As it surrounds internal organs like your kidneys, liver, and pancreas, visceral adipose tissue (VAT), also known as visceral belly fat, is located much lower in your abdomen than subcutaneous fat. This abdominal fat is typically referred to as "harmful."

Visceral fat has a significantly higher metabolic activity than intramuscular fat. The amount of cells, blood vessels, and nerves in this form of fat is higher than in subcutaneous fat.

The hormone insulin, which controls your blood sugar levels, has a stronger association with visceral obesity. Increased blood sugar levels and the onset of type 2 diabetes may occur as a result of insulin resistance over time. The systemic inflammation caused by visceral fat also raises your chance of developing disease.

Men are more likely to acquire an "apple-shaped" figure as belly fat increases because men are more likely than women to accumulate visceral fat. Women, on the other hand, are more likely to accumulate extra body fat in the lower body, giving them a "pear" appearance.

Surprisingly, the spread of body fat alters with age. For instance, while premenopausal women tend to have higher amounts of visceral fat, which raises the risk of metabolic disease, postmenopausal women typically do not.

Additionally, compared to people of other ethnicities, people of European descent tend to have higher levels of visceral fat.

In summary, the soft belly fat that is easy to probe is subcutaneous. Under your skin, it can be discovered. While visceral belly fat encircles the internal organs in your abdominal cavity, there is a clear connection between it and a higher chance of developing disease.

CHAPTER THREE

**I.   WHY HAVING TOO MUCH ABDOMINAL FAT
COULD BE HARMFUL TO YOUR HEALTH**

While having some belly fat is normal and essential for good health, having too much belly fat can be harmful to your well-being and increase your risk of contracting diseases.

The form of belly fat most strongly associated with health issues is visceral fat.

Visceral fat accounts for only 10–20% of the total body fat, but it is closely associated with a higher chance of disease.

This is because visceral fat is "active" fat, which means it creates hormones and other chemicals, such as inflammatory proteins, that are harmful to your health by raising insulin resistance, systemic inflammation, blood fat levels, and blood pressure.

liver and visceral obesity

The portal vein, which carries blood from the gastrointestinal system to the liver for processing, is close to the visceral fat. To your liver, visceral fat transfers fatty acids, inflammatory proteins, and other harmful compounds.

As a result, visceral fat is linked to increased liver fat and liver inflammation, which raises your chance of developing diseases like insulin resistance and nonalcoholic fatty liver disease.

Risk of illness and total abdominal fat

The importance of reducing total belly fat, not just visceral belly fat, cannot be overstated. While subcutaneous belly fat isn't as closely associated with disease risk as visceral fat, having high levels of total belly and body fat is.

According to studies, the buildup of extra body fat plays a significant role in the occurrence of metabolic syndrome, insulin resistance, fatty liver, atherosclerosis (plaque buildup in the arteries), hypertension, and atherosclerosis as well as dysfunction of the blood vessels.

Additionally, research indicates that individuals with more visceral fat have higher risks for several diseases, including type 2 diabetes, metabolic disease, fatty liver, and elevated heart diseases risk factors like high blood pressure and blood fat levels.

Additionally, research involving more than 36,000 individuals discovered that those with higher visceral fat concentrations than subcutaneous fat was more likely to pass away from any cause than those with lower concentrations of visceral fat.

A larger waist circumference is also significantly associated with an increased chance of disease. Waist circumference measures total abdominal fat, so visceral and subcutaneous fat both contribute to this number.

Studies repeatedly demonstrate that a healthy waist circumference can be achieved through nutrition and exercise and that doing so can significantly improve several aspects of health, particularly heart health and diabetes risk.

In summary, there is a direct link between visceral fat and a higher chance of disease. Even though subcutaneous fat isn't thought to be as detrimental as visceral fat, it's crucial to concentrate on decreasing your overall belly fat for the best health.

II. HOW TO REDUCE ABDOMINAL FAT USING PROVEN TECHNIQUES

After learning about the various belly fat types and their effects on your health, you might be wondering how to get rid of extra belly fat in a healthy and long-lasting manner.

Remember that although food and lifestyle have a big impact on belly fat accumulation, other elements like age, sex, and genetics also play a part.

Thankfully, there are several methods to reduce excess belly fat and, consequently, your risk of developing a variety of illnesses.

Here are a few tried-and-true suggestions for reducing abdominal fat:

• **Avoid drinks with added sugar.** Increased visceral fat buildup and a wider waist circumference have both been related to consuming excessive amounts of sugary beverages like soda. Try substituting effervescent water or water for sugary beverages.

• **Start moving.** The amount of exercise you get may help you lose a lot of abdominal fat. A variety of exercises that have been shown to help decrease belly fat include high and moderate-intensity aerobic activity, as well as resistance training.

• **Up your consumption of fiber**. People who consume a diet rich in fiber typically have less belly fat than those who do not. Additionally, switching to a high-fiber diet might help you reduce extra belly fat.

• **Eat less highly processed cuisine.** According to studies, consuming ultra-processed foods frequently, such as fast food, desserts, snacks, and grains made from refined grains, is associated with a larger waist circumference.

• **Drink in moderation**. Alcohol abuse can negatively impact your general health in several ways, including by encouraging an excessive buildup of belly fat.

• **Get enough slumber.** The visceral fat buildup is correlated with poor sleep quality. Additionally, a study involving over 56,000 individuals found a link between increased waist circumference and shorter sleep duration.

• **Up your protein consumption**. Increased protein diets may aid in the reduction of abdominal fat. A study with 23,876 participants found a connection between higher protein diets and a smaller waist circumference. Eat plenty of whole meals. Limiting consumption of highly processed foods in favor of whole, minimally processed foods like vegetables, fruits, nuts, beans, and lean meats and healthy sources of fat and protein may help to improve general health and maintain healthy amounts of belly fat.

In addition to the advice provided above, new research indicates that some individuals with excess belly fat may benefit from reducing their carb consumption.

In a 15-week research of 50 middle-aged overweight or obese individuals, it was discovered that those who were given access to a very low carb, high fat, energy-restricted diet that contained only 5% of calories from carbohydrates lost more visceral and abdominal fat than those who consumed less fat. Interestingly, both diets produced comparable levels of weight loss and body fat reduction, but the low-carb, high-fat diet was more successful at reducing belly fat specifically.

According to additional research, individuals at risk of developing type 2 diabetes and women with the polycystic ovarian syndrome may benefit from reduced visceral fat by restricting their intake of carbohydrates. (PCOS).

However, since diet is highly individualized, some people may experience better results with a higher carbohydrate consumption, especially if those carbs are included in a diet that prioritizes plants and is high in fiber, and includes whole grains, legumes, vegetables, and fruit. (56).

You can make an informed dietary decision that supports reducing belly fat and improving overall health while also catering to your unique requirements and preferences by consulting with a knowledgeable healthcare expert, such as a registered dietitian.

In summary, exercising more, consuming more fiber-rich foods, avoiding sugary drinks and highly processed foods, and getting enough sleep are all tactics for reducing belly fat.

For individualized dietary guidance, you may also want to speak with a registered dietitian.

In conclusion

An increased chance of developing diseases like metabolic disease and fatty liver is one of the negative health effects of having excess belly fat, particularly visceral belly fat.

Luckily, there are lots of healthy methods to losing extra belly fat, such as eating more foods high in nutrients, getting enough sleep, and exercising more.

Aiming for rapid weight loss is not the best strategy for your general health; instead, focus on developing healthy, lifelong habits.

Contact an experienced registered dietitian for more individualized dietary guidance on how to reduce your chance of disease and lose excess belly fat.

CHAPTER FOUR

I. THE BEST WAY TO REDUCE LOWER BELLY FAT

Toning your lower abdomen usually entails losing fat all over your body because you can't usually lose fat from one part of your body at a time. Eating a balanced diet, exercising frequently, drinking plenty of water, and getting enough sleep are a few crucial measures to take to achieve this.

The way each person's body accumulates fat varies. For many individuals, the lower belly is where fat tends to accumulate. This is brought on by genetics, diet, inflammation, and lifestyle variables.

When trying to lose abdominal fat, patience is essential, but there are some things you can do to speed up the process.

Getting rid of belly fat in the bottom third

First, give up the notion that you can "spot treat" fat-filled regions on your body. To tighten your waistline, you can perform countless repetitions of toning movements, but you won't lose fat.

Crunches, yoga, and cardio workouts may help you tone your muscles and strengthen your lower abdomen, but they won't "erase" fat deposits from your body.

Only by losing weight generally will you be able to reduce fat in your lower abdomen. This is facilitated by a calorie shortage.

Creating a calorie imbalance

The key to creating a calorie deficit is a straightforward arithmetic equation: Are you burning more calories each day than you are consuming? In that case, you have a calorie shortage.

The Mayo Clinic states that 3,500 extra calories burned each day equal one pound of fat.

You can shed about 1 pound of fat per week by creating a 500-calorie calorie deficit through diet and exercise.

For the majority of individuals, exceeding 2.5 pounds of fat loss per week necessitates severe calorie restriction and is not advised.

II. HOW TO LOSE EXTRA ABDOMINAL FAT THROUGH DIET

You run the risk of developing visceral fat if you consume more calories than you expend. It can occasionally gather in the area of the belly.

Choosing the proper foods to eat can help you lose weight. Foods that are heavily processed, have a high sugar and grain content and should be avoided or limited. They have been connected to gastrointestinal system inflammation and unstable blood sugar levels.

Instead, concentrate on increasing the amount of wholesome protein and fiber in your food. Cruciferous vegetables are nutrient-rich and may help you feel fuller longer. These include broccoli, kale, and cauliflower.

Without adding many calories to your daily calorie requirements, protein can increase your vitality and stamina. Hard-boiled eggs, lean meats, lentils, and legumes are a few examples of protein sources.

Energy drinks and diet beers among other beverages with artificial sweeteners should be avoided or consumed in moderation. Drink anti-inflammatory drinks only, such as water and unsweetened green tea.

III. HOW TO REDUCE LOWER BELLY FAT THROUGH ACTIVITY

HIIT High-intensity interval training, or HIIT, has been connected to a decrease in fat among heavier people.

In one research, adults who performed three times a week of HIIT exercise experienced outcomes comparable to those of daily 30-minute sessions of moderate cardio. The writers of the study emphasize the importance of long-term regimen adherence for positive outcomes.

To measure your intervals, you can either use an app or a stopwatch. Decide on the activities you'll perform, such as sprints, burpees, speed bag, or another cardio exercise, and work your body as hard as you can for at least 45 seconds.

Take a 45-second break before performing as many repetitions of the exercise as you can in that time. That should be done in a circuit with five to seven movements.

Before performing other exercises, like the ones mentioned below, to burn fat, perform a HIIT or cardio workout.

A great method to intensify your workout is to increase your heart rate before engaging in other forms of physical activity like weightlifting and Pilates.

THREE HIIT EXERCISES FOR THE ARMS AND LEGS

The hundred is a traditional Pilates practice that works the inner deep abs. How to do it is as follows:

1. To begin, lie flat on your back on a yoga cushion with your knees bent and your feet on the ground.

2. Float your legs up one at a time so that your feet are still flexed and your knees are in a tabletop posture.

3. Lift your wrists about an inch off the ground and point your fingers away from you.

4. To activate your abs, raise your upper back and torso off the floor.

5. As you lift your torso and neck off the floor, inhale and start pumping your arms up and down. Start counting while attempting to coordinate your breathing with the motion of your limbs.

6. Remain in the position for a count of 100 before hugging your legs to your chest and exhaling to loosen the tension in your chest. If you can, repeat this exercise two or three times before increasing the number of repetitions.

Scissors Switch

Another lower core exercise that is occasionally used in Pilates exercises is the scissor-switch. This is how you do it:

1. To begin, lie on your back on a yoga mat and raise your legs at a 90-degree angle toward the sky. You should flex your ankles. Your hands can be tucked behind your back.

2. Lift your chin to your torso and maintain the position until your rib cage curves inward toward your belly button. Your lower abdomen should start to contract.

3. Slowly allow one of your legs to descend toward the floor. If you can, halt your leg before it touches the ground and hold it just an inch off the ground.

4. Raise that limb again. As you hold up your chest, repeat with the other limb, alternating. 20 times in total.

Slice with a scalpel

Exercises on the floor that target the lower abdomen include jackknife crunches. After a few repetitions, you'll notice how the action tightens your core even though it initially seems simple.

Here's how to carry them out:

1. In a flat, backward position, stretch for the wall behind you with your arms up over your ears.

2. While focusing on your midsection, raise your arms toward your legs. At the same moment, raise your back and extend your legs toward your head.

3. Touch your legs and then lower your arm.

4. Complete 20 repetitions. Start with three rounds of 20 and increase your reps from there.

Lifestyle adjustments to lose weight

You can alter other aspects of your living in addition to diet and exercise to help you lose weight.

Healthy behaviors frequently cascade into others. If you can incorporate one or two healthy changes into your daily routine, it will get simpler over time to incorporate more.

Here are a few to think about:

• Sip a lot of water.

• Increase the amount of exercise you do each day.

• Try consuming more slowly and with awareness. Slowing down while you consume can prevent you from overeating.

• Give up smoking before attempting any calorie-restricting diet. In addition to the many other health advantages of giving up smoking, it will make your exercises more enjoyable and productive. It can be challenging to stop smoking, but a doctor can assist you in creating a strategy that is ideal for you.

• When you can, get a decent night's sleep. Sleep deprivation has been associated with weight growth and stress increase.

IV. AFTER CHILDBIRTH, HOW TO GET RID OF LOWER ABDOMINAL FAT

Getting your stomach in shape after giving birth could be more difficult. Before beginning any diet or fitness program, wait until your doctor gives the all-clear.

After pregnancy, it's common to have loose skin or an extra layer of fat covering your stomach, particularly if you underwent a cesarean delivery.

Women frequently put on weight while pregnant. You'll probably still have an additional coating of fat on your body after delivery, which you can use as a source of energy for breastfeeding and the healing process after giving birth.

This is a typical component of your body's instinct. It's crucial to have patience with yourself.

In a few instances, you can generally adhere to the same procedures as you did before becoming pregnant to lose postpartum weight.

While nursing, don't limit your calorie intake. Your ability to produce breast milk may be affected.

You might have a disease known as diastasis recti if it appears that pregnancy has torn the muscles in your lower abs apart.

Traditional crunch routines may make it worse. If you think you may have this, talk to your doctor about exercise and physical therapy alternatives.

V. REASONS WHY MEN AND WOMEN BOTH GET ABDOMINAL FAT

The factors behind why you acquire belly fat might be influenced by your sex. Due to hormones, genetics, and aging, women prefer to store belly fat in the lower part of the body, which can be challenging to lose in some situations.

But regardless of sex or gender, everyone should follow the same general strategy for losing weight.

Takeaway

Spot-treating only one region of your body won't help you lose all of the fat there. The only method for safely losing belly fat is to reduce weight overall.

Trimming your waistline can be accomplished by toning and tightening your abs with floor exercises, altering your diet, and establishing healthy practices.

CHAPTER FIVE

I. HOW MUCH TIME WILL IT TAKE ME TO SHED EXTRA BELLY FAT?

Although having some body fat is beneficial, there are valid reasons to want to reduce excess weight around your midsection.

According to Harvard Medical School, the majority of people's body fat is located just below the epidermis. Subcutaneous adipose is what this is.

Visceral fat is the remaining 10% of body fat. It is found in areas near organs and beneath the abdomen walls. That is the fat linked to a variety of illnesses, including type 2 diabetes, heart disease, and cancer.

There is no simple or quick solution if you aim to lose belly fat. Supplements and crash diets are ineffective. Additionally, it's unlikely to focus on reducing fat in just one region of the body.

The ideal strategy for you is to reduce your overall body fat through diet and exercise. There's a good possibility that some of the weight you lose will come from your stomach once you get going.

Each person's experience with that will vary in length. Continue reading to find out how long it usually takes to lose extra belly fat and how to commence.

II. HOW QUICKLY DOES FAT MELT OFF?

To drop 1 pound, you must expend about 3,500 calories. Because 3,500 calories are roughly equivalent to 1 pound of fat.

You must cut 500 calories per day from your diet to drop 1 pound per week. If you continue at that rate, you might drop 4 pounds in a month.

You'll burn more calories if you increase your physical exercise. Muscle bulk is increased through exercise. Even though you feel and appear leaner, the scale may not reflect that because muscle weighs more than fat.

Every person is unique. How much exercise it takes to expend a calorie depends on a variety of factors.

You expend more calories doing anything the bigger you are. Males generally have more muscle than girls of the same size, which increases their calorie expenditure.

How to inflict a calorie deficit?

Energy from sustenance is measured in calories. Calories are burned more quickly the more energy you expend. Fat is the result of unused energy. Fewer calories consumed and increased energy expenditure will help you burn fat reserves.

You can start immediately using these strategies to reduce your caloric intake:

Change beverages

• Choose water over pop.

• Instead of coffee that has been flavored with milk and sugar, try drinking it black.

• Consume less booze.

Steer clear of meals with lots of calories.

• Steer clear of fast cuisine and highly processed foods.

• Opt for fruit instead of packaged sweets and baked products.

• Select low-fat dairy products instead of high-fat ones.

• Opt for grilled or broiled meals rather than fried ones.

• Look up the calorie content on eatery menus. A typical restaurant dinner contains a surprising amount of calories.

• Make use of a free calorie-tracking program.

smaller servings

• Take heating oil measurements.

• Consume fewer vegetable dressings and oils.

• Make use of a tiny plate or bowl.

• Eat more slowly and give yourself 20 minutes to digest.

Avoid eating in front of the TV, where it's simple to keep snacking and take half of your restaurant dinner home.

Also, think about dietary density. For instance, a cup of grapes has approximately 100 calories, whereas a cup of raisins has approximately 480. You can feel full without consuming many calories by eating fresh fruits and veggies because they are high in fiber and water content.

You'll require a lot of protein to maintain lean muscle mass.

20 randomized control trials on diet and weight reduction were the subject of a meta-analysis in 2016 by researchers. They concluded that calorie-restricted, higher-protein diets were more effective at promoting fat loss and maintaining lean mass in people 50 and older than diets with typical protein intakes.

Try these exercises in addition to a normal exercise program:

• Park further away and take the additional distance.

• Rather than driving, you should bike or stroll.

• If possible, take the steps rather than the escalator or elevator.

• After meals, go for a walk.

• Get up from your desk at least once an hour to stretch or take a quick stroll if you work from a desk.

Numerous enjoyable pursuits, including hiking, dancing, and even golfing, help you lose weight. For instance, a 125-pound person can expend 135 calories and a 185-pound person can burn 200 calories in 30 minutes of general gardening.

You burn more calories when you exercise more. And the greater your chances of losing some abdominal fat.

What constitutes success?

To keep note of your overall weight, weigh yourself once a week at the same time of day.

You're likely gaining muscle if you consume a lot of protein and exercise frequently. But keep in mind that the gauge doesn't provide the full picture.

Use a tape measure to determine whether you are truly losing belly fat. Measure in the same spot every time.

Without sucking in your stomach, maintain an upright posture. Avoid pulling the tape so tight that it pinches the flesh. Measure the height of your belly button.

Your garments fitting better and you're beginning to feel better are two additional telltale signs.

exercises for abdominal fat loss

High-intensity intermittent exercise may be more efficient than other forms of exercise at decreasing subcutaneous and abdominal body fat, according to research published in the Journal of Obesity.

Although abdominal exercises may not have an impact on visceral fat, they can strengthen your muscles, which is a positive thing.

It's crucial to stay active and schedule exercise in your day. You are not required to focus exclusively on one subject. So that you don't get tired, vary it. Try performing the following exercises: stretching before bed and in the morning; 30 minutes of moderate-intensity exercise most days; aerobic exercise twice a week; strength training to develop muscle mass.

Takeaway

The optimal strategy might not be to only target belly fat. You must alter your habits to lose weight and keep it off. Start with one small adjustment if it sounds like too much, then add others once you're ready.

Since it's not a "diet," if you relapse, not all is lost. This is a new method of living! Furthermore, it's a wise strategy to move slowly and steadily.

CHAPTER SIX

I. HOW TO REDUCE UPPER BELLY FAT HEALTHILY

Frustration over upper belly fat is prevalent. The best strategy is to exercise to tone your upper belly while working on overall weight reduction.

Where your body stores excess fat is influenced by a combination of genetics, living choices, and dietary habits. For some individuals, fat loss happens last in the upper belly area.

A layer of fat might still be present even after activity. However, it can be decreased with a combination of cardio exercise, weight training, weight reduction, and lifestyle choices.

To get you begun, consider the following steps.

How to get rid of the upper abdominal fat

In some crucial respects, upper belly fat differs from lower belly fat. It is more difficult to lose lower abdominal fat because it is slightly less absorbable. But upper abdominal fat can also be difficult to lose.

There is no truth to the notion that you can target particular fat stores in your body with exercise. Without losing body fat overall, you cannot reduce fat in any one region of your body.

Your plan will generally include the same elements: calorie restriction, weight training, and lifestyle modifications, regardless of how much weight or fat you're attempting to lose.

Recognize that having some body fat is healthy, normal, and a necessary component of being a human before you attempt to decrease it. Losing upper abdominal fat may be particularly difficult and time-consuming if your body mass index (BMI) is already low.

How to reduce calories consumed?

You need to comprehend the fundamental idea before you can produce a caloric deficit. Unless you have an underlying health condition that affects your weight, your weight will stay fairly stable if the number of calories you consume each day and the number of calories you expend through exercise are equal.

You need to eat fewer calories than you burn each day if you want to drop weight or reduce body fat. You can achieve this by cutting back on your daily caloric consumption, increasing your level of daily activity, or doing both.

You must expend an additional 3,500 calories through a caloric deficit to lose one pound of fat. You will lose weight at a pace of about one pound per week if you consistently burn 500 more calories per day than you take in.

It is not advised for most people to lose more than 1.5 to 2 pounds per week because doing so necessitates excessive calorie reduction.

diet to reduce fat in the upper abdomen

When attempting to lose weight, what you consume is important. There are a few crucial things to bear in mind when dieting to lose upper belly fat.

Your body may retain water, which can lead to upper abdominal fat. Your body may hold water if you consume too much sodium, become dehydrated, or don't get enough electrolytes.

As a result, your body parts may look swollen, including your stomach. Whenever you're trying to reduce belly fat, keep to a low-salt diet.

How much fiber you consume can have an impact on belly obesity as well. When you're not consuming enough fiber, your stomach can be pushed outward by gases and waste in your digestive system.

The cause of this is a slow-moving digestive system that lacks sufficient fiber to expeditiously move food through and out of your digestive tract.

Consequently, consuming a diet rich in fiber-rich foods can aid in the reduction of belly fat and overall weight gain. Additionally, fiber helps you feel fuller for longer, which makes calorie counting simpler.

Avoid white starches, processed grains, soft drinks, and sugar-rich foods when trying to reduce belly fat. Your endocrine system may be disturbed by these meals, which also makes it more difficult for your body to burn fat.

II. HOW TO WORK YOUR WAY OUT OF EXTRA BELLY FAT

While you're trying to lose weight, these activities will help to strengthen your core, tone your waist, and improve your posture. However, they won't help to "spot treat" areas of fat on your body.

Share the boat image on Pinterest

Start easy with Boat Pose if you want to try yoga for weight reduction.

1. Extend your legs out in front of you as you sit on a yoga cushion.

2. With your legs flexed, raise your feet off the ground until your shins are parallel to the surface.

3. Extend as far as you can with your knees while extending your arms in front of you.

4. While maintaining awareness of your respiration, hold the position for at least 30 seconds.

5. Get your core and upper abdomen in gear by returning to a neutral position and repeating 8–10 times.

Russian gimmicks

Despite how easy this exercise is; after just a few repetitions you'll start to feel the burn in your upper abdomen. To make this more difficult, add weights or a medicine ball.

1. Sit on a yoga mat with your feet flat, your legs bent, and your butt on the floor.

2. With your abdominal tightened and your butt firmly planted on the floor, sag back until your back is at a 45-degree angle with the ground.

3. Squeeze your hands together just above your belly button. Bring your weight over to the affected side of your body by slowly rotating it to that side.

4. Turn around and face the opposite direction. If you sense that your equilibrium is slipping, cross your ankles.

5. If you can, rapidly rotate your body in both directions while keeping your legs at a 45-degree angle.

6. Strive to maintain your momentum for a complete minute before stopping.

ascending plank

The deep transverse abdominal muscles, which are simple to overlook during workouts, are targeted by this activity to tone your upper belly.

1. Lie flat on your back with your legs straight out in front of you and your arms erect, palms down.

2. Squeeze your abs and picture a cord connected to your belly button pulling you upward. Pushing up from the belly, using your hands. Attempt to climb higher by wearing shoes.

3. After sustaining this posture for a few seconds, release it and smoothly revert to the neutral position. For a single performance, repeat 10–12 times.

A side plank

Both your obliques and upper abdomen are worked out by these planks.

One arm should be extended as you lie supine on one side. Make a 45-degree angle with your thighs while bending your knees.

2. Support your weight by placing your outstretched arms and forearm on the ground. Get into a sideways plank posture by pulling in your oblique muscles.

3. Raise the arm that isn't touching the ground toward the sky, and maintain this posture for as long as you can.

4. Make a slow spin around and get back to where you were. For a single performance, repeat 8–10 times.

III. CHANGING YOUR WAY OF LIFE TO LOSE WEIGHT

There are other decisions you can make to help decrease belly fat besides exercising and calorie counting.

water intake

For some individuals, drinking water facilitates weight reduction. Additionally, it lessens inflammation, enhances digestion, hydrates muscles for improved workout efficiency, and removes toxins from your body.

lower your tension level

Even if you're following all the right procedures to reduce weight, stress may be the cause of stubborn fat deposits.

Try stress-relieving techniques like yoga, deep breathing, and mindfulness even though you might not be able to eliminate tension from your life. All of these also have the benefit of making weight reduction simpler.

Make a strategy for quitting smoking.

If you smoke, quitting might initially feel like it makes you acquire weight as you struggle to control your cravings for nicotine. But after quitting, you'll probably find it simpler to get active and lose weight. Additionally, you'll be considered healthy.

Although it can be difficult to stop smoking, you can develop a personalized strategy with the help of your doctor.

What results in belly fat gain?

Typically, eating more calories than you burn off is the primary contributor to abdominal weight gain. It's not quite that easy, though. In addition to hormones, aging, menopause, lack of sleep, genetics, and stress, other factors can contribute to fat buildup in the upper belly region.

Takeaway

Your muscles will become stronger and more toned by working out your upper body and spine, but the layer of belly fat cannot be "spot-treated."

The only way to get rid of belly fat deposits is to create a plan to reduce weight generally. This might be difficult for some individuals who don't need to drop a lot of weight.

When deciding how fast to lose weight, try to be realistic. Keep in mind that fat is a component of all bodies and that it is not always a reliable sign of your level of health.

Consult a doctor to establish healthy weight reduction goals appropriate for your height and body type if you're worried about fat in your upper abdomen.